Running Reaper

Poems from an Impatient Cancer Survivor

Running from the Reaper
Poems from an Impatient Cancer Survivor

John Smelcer

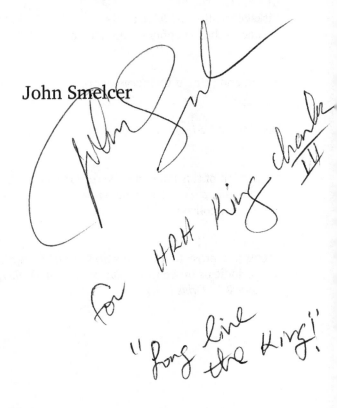

For HRH King Charles III
"Long live the King!"

Leap Faith Press
Kirksville, Missouri

Running from the Reaper © 2023 John Smelcer
Cover illustration © 2023 John Smelcer
Cover design by Rusty Nelson.

ISBN   978-1-0879-0815-1

Leap Faith Press
813 E. Harrison St.
Kirksville, Missouri 63501 USA
Contact: johnsonamber8@gmail.com

Bound and printed by IngramSpark

Distributed by Ingram Booksellers

Poems and prose in this collection originally appeared in the following periodicals or websites: Oncolink, *Cure Today, Conquer, Coping, Curiosus* & in *Orbis* (UK).

"Run away! We must run away. It's him. [Death]"
–Leo Tolstoy's last words

"No one here gets out alive."
–Jim Morrison, of The Doors

Books by John Smelcer

Fiction
The Trap, Kiska, Stealing Indians, Savage Mountain,
Edge of Nowhere, Lone Wolves, The Great Death

Native Studies
The Raven and the Totem, Trickster
A Cycle of Myths, In the Shadows of Mountains
The Day That Cries Forever, Native American Classics
We are the Land, We are the Sea

Poetry
Raven, Indian Giver, Durable Breath,
The Indian Prophet, Songs from an Outcast, Riversong,
Without Reservation, Tracks, Raven Speaks,
Beautiful Words: The Complete Ahtna Poems

Nonfiction
Enacting Love: How Thomas Merton Died for Peace
A New Day: Meditations to Inspire Compassion

Contents

*for my wife and daughters, with hope that
I might dwell in their lives for years to come.*

INTRODUCTION

Let me say from the start that this is a book I never would have expected to write or hoped to write in all my life. But once it began, the poems came out of me faster than anything I've ever experienced. It was magic. Or maybe it was medicine. The poems were necessary, the way good poetry is always necessary. This book began because of three simple words: "You have cancer."

In the fall of 2022, my life was changed by a single phone call when I was diagnosed with stage 2 B-cell, non-specified, non-Hodgkin's Lymphoma, a rare and aggressive cancer of the lymphatic system. For me, a large tumor was growing in my left armpit. The tumor was damaging my ulnar nerve to the point that for more than a year my pinky and closest finger always hurt with a painful electric shock that never went away. I also lost feeling and most the use of both fingers. As the mass grew, the pain and intensity increased. One local doctor thought it was a simple case of nerve impingement, something, perhaps in my elbow, was constricting the nerve and causing the pain. Another thought it was arthritis and gave me an anointment. Another thought it was related to my weightlifting in the gym, so he told me to stop lifting heavy weights. Finally, after seeing three different local doctors who kept misdiagnosing my condition, I was referred to a specialist in a larger city who in short order ordered an MRI, a biopsy, and a PET scan. Within days, I was told that I had cancer and that I would be dead in three months if I did nothing. From that moment, I began my arduous journey down the foot-worn path trod by many before me, asking questions such as "Why me?" and "What did I do to deserve getting cancer?

Fortunately, I was told that my cancer was curable with chemotherapy and immunotherapy. But because of the nature and the size of the tumor, my treatment had to be immediate and aggressive—only the strongest chemo would knock down the cancer. Days after receiving the diagnosis, I was admitted to the Ellis Fischel Cancer Center at MU Health in Columbia, Missouri. For the next half year, I spent a week in the hospital every month in the very capable hands of doctors, nurses, radiologists, techs, and other staff. During that time, my own mortality was never far from my thoughts. All I had to do was to look in the mirror to see death lurking over my shoulder. Fortunately, the cancer responded positively to the chemo. A second PET scan between the third and fourth cycle revealed that the tumor was totally gone. I was, in effect, cancer-free. But, to be safe, I'd have to endure a few more cycles of chemo to make sure the lymphoma did not return or manifest elsewhere in my body. To prevent it from lodging in my brain, I endured numerous intrathecal injections of a specialized chemo into my lower spinal disks.

The subtitle of this book, *Poems from an Impatient Cancer Survivor*, comes from my reluctance to undergo my sixth and final treatment. After five cycles of chemotherapy, I was sick and tired of the hospitalizations and my body's rollercoaster ride of ruin and recovery. I argued fervently with the chief oncologist to let me be done. I implored him, "Is there any medical evidence that six cycles is significantly better than five?" Fortunately, cooler heads prevailed and I completed all six cycles (mostly for my family's sake)

I am happy to say that on an unseasonably warm day in early February 2023, I got to "Ring the Bell" on the Oncology ward, signaling the successful completion of my cancer treatment. The long road of recovery lay ahead of me

Instead of maintaining a journal, I decided from the day I received my diagnosis to write down my thoughts, concerns, fears, experiences, and tribulations as poetry. After all—as I often remind my students—the sheer act of writing poetry is the compulsion to express ourselves, even in, and especially in the face of our own demise. As best I could, I have arranged the poems chronologically to tell the story as it unfolded. They say no two cancer patients go through the grueling process in the exact same way. There are numerous chemotherapy regiments and protocols, reactions, including allergic reactions—some severe. Fortunately, I had no adverse reactions. Some patients undergo chemo once a week for a few hours in Ambulatory Infusion. Others, like me, spent five days at a time in the hospital because the chemotherapy was so aggressive, so poisonous. Finally, there are desirable and undesirable outcomes. Many patients go into remission; others do not. But the similarities of the treatments and emotions we all experience are enough that this book may have some worth and be of some help.

Two months after I rang the bell, according to protocol, I had a follow-up PET scan to make sure the cancer hadn't returned. I'm happy to say the results were negative—nothing suspicious was detected. My cancer is gone. The only trace that it ever existed is these poems.

Running from the Reaper

ON RECEIVING RESULTS OF A BIOPSY

"Cancer," she said before hanging up.
And just like that my world was shattered.

A single word,
the one they told me I probably wouldn't hear.

"If it was cancer," the previous doctors had said,
"it would be bigger by now and you'd be in more pain."

But they were wrong. They were all wrong.
The woman on the phone said it was aggressive.
I didn't like the sound of that.

For a long time I sat with the phone in my lap,
stunned, mumbling the word over and over,
each time the word becoming more real, concrete—
my future less certain, as if I was standing before a cavern.
For the first time in my life, I understood
the way Noah must surely have stopped his labor
from time to time, wiped his sweaty brow,
and gazed fretfully at the dark, roiling clouds.

A GRIMM FAIRY TALE

News of my cancer diagnosis
cast me into a forest, deep and dark—

the kind in fairy tales

where ominous trees lunge to snatch me in their boughs,
where bats flutter in the moonless sky,
and yellow eyes and eerie shrieks pierce the gloom.

Now I know how Hansel and Gretel must have felt
as they strew bread crumbs along the way.

I pull my collar up against the cold and damp,
lean into the blasting gale, and push on warily.

Death is my companion now.
There's no time to linger, no safe haven.
For the woods are deep and dark,
and there are many miles to go before I can stop to rest.

SURVIVOR MAN

In my life I've survived

a bear attack,

a wolf attack

and a bull moose that nearly drowned me

when it dragged me across a river while sleeping in my tent.

I survived falling into a glacial crevasse

by clawing my way out with pitons;

and my brother and I once almost slid off a mountain.

How bad can cancer be compared to what I've already been through?

I tell you, cancer ain't near as scary as that bear and them wolves.

MY BODY, MY ENEMY

All my life I've taken care of you.
I started weight-lifting in junior high;
competed internationally through two decades.
Never drank a beer until I was 30;
never smoked a joint or cigarette.
Ate balanced meals with vegetables. Vegetables!
Cut out candy-ass kid's breakfast cereals and fast foods.
Always said no to drugs the way that TV commercial
with the hot frying pan and a sizzling egg taught me.

My doctor used to say I was the fittest older man he'd ever seen.

But none of that mattered.
Instead, you repay me with cancer,
the way one of my old girlfriends blindsided me
when she stole all my money and took off to Spain
with her new Latin lover.

THAT WHICH MUST NOT BE NAMED

Like every person throughout history
I ask, "Why me?" "Why did I get cancer?"
"What did I do to deserve this, to deserve *It*?"
"How is this possible?"
                    And yet *It* is.

I run from *It*, ignore *It*, rail at *It*, and pound my fists against *It*.

But every time I look in a mirror I'm face-to-face with *It* –
                    and cannot deny *It*,

this thing staring dumbly back at me as I shudder in horror.

ROAD MAP

I never thought I'd get cancer.
Over and over, I said to myself:

"I shouldn't be here. I should be somewhere else.
What am I doing here? How did I get to this place?"

At one time or another
we each pull out the tattered map of our lives
carefully unhinge the torn and ragged folds
press it flat on a table with both hands like an iron
lean over and trace its topography with a finger
frantically searching for the familiar X that says

You Are Here

THE FIGHTER

Folks always say that people diagnosed with cancer are "fighters."
"He's fighting cancer," they say.

But I'm not so sure.

I just finished my second cycle of chemo—
a week in the hospital both times.
I'm no fighter. I'm a *surrenderer.*

I just lie in bed giving in to the cure
letting the doctors and nurses put whatever they want into me:

>Hang another bag of chemo,
>
>swallow a heap of pills,
>
>roll over for a spinal infusion.

"We're killing you to save you," they remind me every day.
And they're not lying. I've lost ten pounds already.
All muscle.

I'm no fighter.
I'm just a little, frail, balding, and frightened old man
lying in my sick bed waving a little white flag

>torn from my pillow.

DYLAN THOMAS
WAS TOO YOUNG TO KNOW
WHAT HE WAS TALKING ABOUT

I've always loved Dylan Thomas's

"Do Not Go Gentle into That Good Night,"

his poem in which he urges his dying father

not to give in to death but to fight it every inch

of the way like a madman.

But I was young then, high school and college age.

I thought I'd live forever—a hundred years, for sure.

But near sixty and diagnosed with cancer,

Dylan's poem falls flat on its face.

Everything passes.   Everyone dies.

What good is it to rage against the inescapable?

Even the stars one day burn out and die.

WHAT MY MOTHER
SAID ON LEARNING I HAD CANCER

My mother, who suffers from severe dementia,
has been living in a nursing home for two years.

She's always saying hurtful things to me.
Wise friends remind me:

"Don't feel so bad when she says terrible things to you.
Remember, because of the dementia
she is not the person you used to know."

But it's hard not to feel bad
when she says some of the things she says.
Like the time I told her I have a rare and aggressive cancer
and that my doctors told me I could be dead in three months.

But instead of saying she was sorry and hugging me
with tears in her eyes—me her only child—
my mother looked at me blankly and said,

"Before you die, can you bring me my ID card,
passport, credits cards, ATM card, and a suitcase
so I can get out of this joint?"

BENADRYL DELIRIUM

First time they hung a IV bag of Retuxan,
(the name of the immunotherapy part of my chemo)
they pushed in a heavy dose of liquid Benadryl.
(They said it was in case I had an allergic reaction.)

Slowly, I slid into a warm sea of numbness.
But in moments, I felt the most opposite feelings ever
in a single body: On the one hand, I wanted to sleep
as long as Rip Van Winkle, but my jittery, restless legs
wanted to run the Boston Marathon.
Worse Jimmy Legs ever. Sleep or run.

As the sloshing wave washed over me,
I looked over at my wife who had turned the most radiant yellow
I've ever seen. Every bit of her exposed skin was neon yellow.

She could see my bewilderment and incredulity.
I remember the look on her face as I stared agog:
"What?" She said. *"Is there something on my face?"*

ROLLY POLEY

I've become rather attached to my IV pole—
you know the rolling metal thingamajig that hospital patients
push sadly about as they shamble down the hallway
with swinging bags dangling from the hooks.

I named mine Rolly; rhymes with goalie.
(One patient I met calls his Steely Dan.)

They say dogs are man's best friend,
but I don't know about that anymore.
Rolly is such a good boy. He follows every command:

Sit, boy! Stay. Heel.

Rolly always waits patiently by my side.
He loves to go on walks. He follows me everywhere.
And he always comes a running when I call.
"Here, Boy! Heel! Good boy."

Better yet, I never have to feed him,
and I never have to pick up his poo.

IRONY

The doctors and nurses who swap out my chemo bags
and suit up in protective Hazmat gowns and gloves and face shields
before they pump a gallon of that poison into my naked veins.

FALSE PRIDE
ON THE ONCOLOGY WARD

One morning, halfway through my first chemo cycle,
the oncology doctors and a gaggle of gawking residents
visit me in my room.

They ask how I'm feeling, if I have any pain or allergies.
I tell them I'm allergic to work. They all laugh.

I respond, "My body's strong. I feel good enough
to run a marathon." The docs raise their eyebrows.
They know what's coming.

I tell them, "My body can take whatever you dish you out.
I'll sail right through, no problem."
A resident raises his hand to stifle a giggle.

"Nope," I say, "these chemo cycles won't affect me one bit."
As they walk away, I hear the doctor's laughing
all the way down the hall.

CHURROS WITH DEATH

A week after doctors told me I had cancer,
Death came to visit me.

"Is it time already?" I asked, rubbing my sleepy eyes.
"Soon," he muttered. "Soon. Take my hand. Come with me."

Next thing I knew, we were standing in a desert
at a Mexican food truck, ordering churros.

"This is one of the best churros I've ever had," said Death
after taking a bite. "Try it," he said,
pointing at mine with a bony finger.

Thinking he seemed amicable enough, I asked
"Can I have just a little more time?"

Death laughed and slapped his knee.
"You don't know how many billions of times
I've heard that before. Ha! That never gets old!"

As he scurried away, Death turned, waved, and shouted,
"I'll be seeing you around, Johnny Boy!"

CHEMO CYCLE BLUES,
PART I

I was brushing my teeth this morning
when I looked up after spitting.

There in the mirror was a bald man
holding a toothbrush, his eyes
full of bewilderment and incredulity,

his face pallid and gaunt,
his eyes deeply sunken, lips chapped,
his beard and hair gone.

I leaned closer to the glass to better glimpse
the stranger holding my toothbrush.

THE DAY MY HAIR
FELL OUT

Third chemo cycle did the trick.
One day hair; next day bare.

I hoped I'd look like a bad-ass:
Telly Savalas or Yul Brynner or Vin Diesel.

Heck I'd have settled for buff Mr. Clean
with his one shiny gold earring.

Instead, with my wrinkly head and squinty vision
I look more like Mr. Magoo.

THINGS I MISS SINCE
I STARTED CHEMOTHERAPY

Not having a perpetually runny nose

Not swallowing a bucket of pills every day

Pants that don't fall down all the time

      My libido

      My hair

My muscles, my confidence, my stamina

My courage (I'm afraid all the time)

My assured stride, instead of shuffling like the living dead

Being content with my reflection in the mirror

Not thinking about dying all the time

      My libido

      My hair   (everywhere)

CANCER WEIGHT LOSS
COMMERCIAL

Want to shed those unwanted pounds,

but don't have time for the gym?

Try our new Cancer Weight Loss Program!

Lose ten, fifteen, even twenty percent of your body weight!

Be amazed at how fast fat melts and muscles waste away!

Be astonished at how quickly your face looks drawn like a corpse!

      For a limited time only!

      Don't delay! Order today!

      Guaranteed or your money back!

Order now and receive our Hair Loss Program absolutely free!

CHEMO CYCLE BLUES, PART II

Doctors said they wanted to up the dose of my chemo.
"We must try to kill you to save you," they reminded me.

The stronger dose shut down my immune system
So that I was ogled by every passing germ, bacteria, or virus,
the way prostitutes beckon solicitously to sailors

passing a brothel.

All the fast-growing cells in my mouth died.
My tongue was white and blistered.
For days, eating anything was torture.
The pain shot up my ears whenever I chewed,
so I drank those crappy booster drinks instead.

Did I tell you this was all during Thanksgiving?

So much delicious food
that hurt me too much to eat a bite of it,
except for a slice of homemade pumpkin pie
with whipped cream.

(Some things are worth the pain.)

CHEMO BRAIN
(IT'S A THING)

Usually after my second or third bag of chemo
I get Chemo Brain. Some people call it Chemo Fog.

Everything becomes fuzzy and foggy and disconnected.
I can't focus. My vision gets blurred.
I can't recall words easily and I can't type a sentence
withowt tie ping tuns uv typors.

This is all very bad for a poet and a writer.
(I should have been a *Gigolo*.)

Even my walking is affected.
I'm wobbly, off-balanced, uncertain, as if I'm teetering
on a tightrope above the lion cage without a balancing pole.

Going up and down stairs is a challenge.
(I've tripped a few times. Please don't tell my wife.)
The good news is it doesn't usually last longer than a week.

I wish you sunny, fog-free days full of blue skies and sunshine.

THE SNOT KING

At the meeting where the nurse told us
about all the possible side effects of chemo
(the list filled a sheet of paper and included death)
one of the things listed was "runny nose."

What an understatement!
It should have been printed in oversized, bolded font.

Ever since I began chemo my nose runs all the time,
like a leaky faucet or Niagra Falls. It never ends.

There are boxes of tissue in every room of our house.
I go through two or three boxes a day—
that's 2,000 tissues a week; 8,000 a month;
50,000 from beginning to end.

I go through so many tissues that I bought stock in Kleenex.

The price of the stock sky-rocketed from the high demand.
Now I'm a millionaire! I'm the Snot King!

THE CREMATION
OF SAM MCGEE & ME

After the third chemo cycle, I was freezing all the time.

I piled under blankets, took saunas at the YMCA,

but 170 degrees just wasn't hot enough to thaw me.

I was so cold that during Thanksgiving in Tennessee, I swear

I thought about crawling into the oven with the turkey to get warm.

The cozy thought reminded me of a poem by Robert Service,

the famous Gold Rush poet who wrote, "The Cremation of Sam

McGee,"

about a fella' from Tennessee who was cremated

in a red-hot woodstove after freezing to death in the Yukon.

As the poem goes, after a while, his fellow miner opened the door:

"There sat Sam, looking cool and calm

in the heart of the furnace roar;

and he wore a smile you could see a mile,

and he said, "Please close that door.

It's fine in here, but I greatly fear

you'll let in the cold and storm.

Since I left Plumtree, down in Tennessee,
it's the first time I've been warm."

MAN'S BEST FRIEND

My Black Lab is the same age as I am.
(In dog years, that is.)

By the strangest coincidence
We both got tumors at the same time.

Mine's an inconspicuous lymphoma under my armpit.
My dog's is on his ass, big as day.

The vet even had to shave his butt.
Guess I should be thankful for the little things.

IVAN ILYICH SUCKS AS
READING IN A CANCER WARD

I took a book to read in the hospital while undergoing chemo.

I love Tolstoy, so I grabbed *The Death of Ivan Ilyich*,
considered one of the greatest novels ever written.

But as I began to read, I immediately regretted the decision.
I imagined the story was about some Russian political dissident
sent off to a gulag in Siberia who dies of frostbite and starvation.

Instead, it's a dreary and terrifying glimpse
of a man slowly dying from pancreatic cancer
as he stares into the abyss of death and confronts
his own mortality.

It is my story. It is my lot.
I am Ivan Ilyich, only a few years older than he was.
The story does not end well for Ivan Ilyich.
It did not end well for Tolstoy either. In 1910,
he was found dead on a cot in a remote railroad station
in Russia. His last muttered words were:
"Run away! We must run away. It's him, Death."

I hope I fare better, but I'm not so sure.

Only time will tell.

"What do I have to fear," I ask myself.

"Me," Death murmurs from the darkness.

SOLDIER IN A FOXHOLE

I never worried about dying from my cancer
as much as I do now that I can see the light at the end of the tun-
   nel.

Even though the tumor has been gone for months
it's the continued chemo that scares me.

I keep thinking about what the doctors always tell me,
"We're killing you to save you."

As the accumulating effects of the chemo keep getting worse—
taking my body longer and longer to recover each cycle—
the danger of dying seems greater than ever.

Now I know how a short-timer soldier in a muddy foxhole
must feel during a firefight with his separation orders
folded neatly in his pocket, worrying that today
is the day he finally buys the farm.

THE LAST TEAM
BUILDING EXERCISE

I admit I get pretty low in the hospital sometimes.
Oh, I never let on my true feelings. No nurse or doctor
would tell you that they thought I was ever sad.

I put on a good show.

"We love your exuberance!" they tell me time and again
as they pat me on the back.

"We wish every patient had your positive attitude," they say.

But when I look back on my life, I feel as though
I failed at so many things in my life:

being a good husband;
being a good father;
having a successful career.

Honestly, at times I think it might not be so bad to just let go.
I'm not talking about suicide or anything like that.

After so many punishing cycles of chemo and spinal infusions,
I'm talking about letting go with dignity and grace,

about acceptance and trust, as you fall backward
blindly into the awaiting arms of death.

A CANCER PATIENT'S CHRISTMAS PRAYER

This Christmas, I don't care about
a stuffed stocking hanging on the fireplace mantle
or colorful gifts piled beneath the tree.

What I really want is for this tumor to go away.
Let it never come back.
Let me live to accomplish some dreams.
Let me love and be loved.

I still have things I want to do,
places to go,
plans to complete
and new friends to meet.

Some things in life matter more
only when faced with losing them forever.

HOW THE SWEDISH SUPERBAND ABBA REINFORCED MY DESIRE TO LIVE

I never wept for having cancer. Not once.

My wife bawled when the oncologist delivered my diagnosis.

My mother-in-law sobbed when she heard the news.

Heck, I didn't even cry when the doctors said the tumor was gone.

But, standing in the brightening light

near the end of the tunnel, I finally broke down.

Relieved, I wept grateful tears of joy

like the time I saw *Mama Mia!* in a movie theatre.

Watching the musical again tonight reminded me

how much I want to love, laugh, sing, dance, and dream.

I want to feel! I want to be! I want to live!

MESSAGE IN A BOTTLE

One day after the fifth cycle, I was certain I was going to die.
The chemo was killing me, just like my doctors said it would.

I wanted to leave a farewell message for my wife and daughter,
so I recorded a video. In it, I look like an exhumed corpse.

In the video, I apologized for leaving them so soon.

I said I'm sorry I'm gone. I didn't want it to be this way.
I'm sorry you will spend the rest of your lives without me.
I'd have given anything for it to be otherwise.
But I'm glad it was me, not you. You will endure.

I ended the message with the only gift I could muster,
the necessary things I have learned about life:
Pursue joy. Cherish every moment. Love and be loved.

A POET'S LAST WILL & TESTAMENT

I, a poet diagnosed with cancer, being of sound mind
but not of sound body, do hereby bequeath to the world
the following in the event of my untimely demise:

For those without kindness,

    I leave my compassion.

To those who cannot see the pain & suffering of others,

    I leave my empathy.

For those who only see the differences between us,

    I bestow tolerance.

For those who are selfish & greedy,

    I give to you my charity.

To they who are miserly with their time,

    I will my volunteerism.

To those who fail to see the humanity & dignity in every person,

    I leave you my unshakable & selfless love for others.

To those who are in despair,

    I give you my steadfast hope.

To the dejected & downhearted,

    I give you my cheerfulness & joy.

To anyone who lacks vision,

    I give you my imagination & creativity.

For anyone I have ever hurt,

    I express my sincere apology.

For anyone who has been hurt by others,

    I give my forgiveness.

To the unfortunate who have been bullied,

    I leave my integrity & tenacity.

To those who are weary & exhausted,

    I leave my boundless stamina.

To those who are weak,

    I give you my strength.

For those who are lost,

    I leave my sense of direction.

To the lonely,

    I confer the healing power of solitude & silence.

To those full of self-importance,

    I impart my humility.

For those without pity or clemency,

    I give you my mercy.

To those who are without love in their life,

    I give you all my love.

For those who want to be closer to God,

    Love everything & everyone all the time & all at once.

For all those who cannot see the beauty in this world,

I leave my poet's heart.

To those who wish me dead,

    I bequeath my sympathy.

There is nothing else for me to give, nothing else to leave.

    Nothing material matters.

SPINAL TAP

Twice a week, while I was in the hospital
I went down to Radiology for an intrathecal
to inject chemo into my spinal disk.

The first time, they tried to do it in my hospital room
while like half a dozen med students grimaced
and wrung their fretful hands as they watched the doc
unsuccessfully try a dozen times to give me a spinal tap.
But he couldn't get the angle right, so the needle struck bone.
Frustrated, the doctor announced it wasn't going to work.

Over the next four months, I did eight spinal taps in Radiology
where the x-ray machine precisely guided the needle.

They say misery loves company.
I hope this poem made you squirm and your sphincter twitch.

RUFFLES HAVE RIDGES

and so do my fingernails

You know how you can tell the age of a tree
by counting its rings? Each ring is a year.
From their spacing, you can tell how some years were better than
others.
Because of the chemo, my fingernails tell a similar story.

There are five ridges on each nail, which look like
a series of sand dunes or the way high tides are marked
by a waterline on the beach, full of flotsam and foam.
Some might even describe them as ribbed like a rubber.

Doctors call them "Beau's Lines."

Each ridge sheds light on the history between chemo cycles,
when the toxic chemo stopped the nails from growing for a while.
The dune closest to each fingertip was made after the first cycle,
five months ago. Five cycles; five ridges.

My wife, the archaeologist, says my teeth will also show evidence
of the toll the chemo took on my body.

On the list of possible side effects the nurse warned us about
sand dune fingernails were never mentioned.

DASH AWAY ALL

Chemo makes most cancer patients nauseous.
Not so much for me. I puked a couple times
after the first cycle, but never again.

What always brought me closest was the moment I'd lift the lid
that covered every meal ever brought to me in the hospital.
No matter what it was, I almost hurled just looking at it.

Early on, my nurses warned me that if I didn't eat enough
the doctors might order feeding tubes.

So that I wouldn't have tubes shoved down my gullet,
I started to throw the food away into a garbage bag,
tie it off, and dump it in another garbage can
somewhere else in the building.

But I didn't starve. At first, I brought my own food.
Eventually, I got the Door Dash app, which I could use to order
food from my favorite restaurants and have it delivered.
Sometimes, it's the little things that keep you going.

MY WIFE'S SUPERPOWER

Everyone going through cancer should have someone like my wife.

She has no giant gold letter on a tight blue or red shirt
concealed beneath her street clothes waiting for an emergency.

Her superpower is Organization, which is a good thing
during my cancer treatment, because she took all the calls
from the oncology clinic, managed all my appointments,
refilled every prescription, got me to where I was supposed to be,
and drove me home when I was exhausted and chemo-brained
from each boring-ass hospital stay. She gathered all the statements
from the hospital and insurance, paid the bills, and filed the forms
away in a cabinet like nobody's business.

But she'd tell you her real superpower was her love for me.

Look there, soaring high above that skyscraper!
It's not a bird or a plane.

It's my wife riding her magic, flying ten-key calculator

with her cell phone in one hand and daily planner in the other—

the long, white, paper tape

    fluttering

      like

        a

          kite tail.

ELVIS HAS LEFT
THE BUILDING

Three things to tell you first:

> My middle name is Elvis.
>
> I've always been a rebel.
>
> My hospital room was the nicest you ever saw.

But a cage gilded with gold is still a prison.
For me, I could never stand a cubicle job
or one in a small office. I feel imprisoned.
Raised in the wilds of Alaska, I need the freedom
of   wide   open   spaces.

I would have tied bedsheets together and rappelled
out the eight-story window if they gave me enough sheets.

Instead, for six months, I snuck out from the Oncology floor
half a dozen times a day. My great escape didn't include
jumping over a barbwire fence on a motorcycle.

> It was more devious than that.

I'd shuffle out to the elevator lobby with my IV poll
and act nonchalant like I was looking at a magazine
or the vending machine until the nurse at the desk

was distracted, then I'd push the button

and take the elevator anywhere but there.

Sometimes, when the nurses were waiting

for the next chemo bag to come up from pharmacy

(which sometimes took two or three hours)

I'd sneak past security at the main door

and leave the building entirely, walking blocks away,

ducking into coffee houses, a grocery, a record shop, and a bakery.

To aid my duplicity, I never wore those back-and-ass-baring

hospital gowns. I always wore my street clothes

so folks wouldn't know I was a patient.

It felt good to be seen as normal, even if only for a spell.

For those brief but cherished escapes,

I was free of my cancer, free of my fear.

THE GOOD, THE BAD,
AND THE UGLY

I will never forget how I was blinded
by the way my wife looked at me as we exchanged our vows—
the way she looked right through me, her gaze
more powerful than anything I had ever known,
like staring at the sun.

"For better or for worse,
through sickness and in health,
through good times and bad times . . ."

That's what the preacher said.

When my wife married me she got them all:

Worse, sickness, hard times.

There's been good times, for sure.
More than I deserve.

I have two wonderful daughters who love me,
two dogs that think I'm the cat's meow,
(though the cat would beg to differ)
and in-laws who generally think I'm good enough
for their daughter

(she deserves better).

I couldn't ask for more.

(Could you?)

But the past six months of cancer and chemo and uncertainty
have taken their toll on all of us.

What have I learned from it all?

That my wife loves me to the moon, and I love her
to the moon and back (and then some).
It's been said in so many ways over so many years,
"Love conquers all."

I have no doubt that the love in my life conquered everything
that hurled and battered itself against it.

FRIGHT NIGHT

I am surrounded by death and dying.

Whenever I stroll around the Oncology floor
I see the terminally-ill patients sunken in their beds.
I suppose they are the more grave Stage IV cases.
(I've since learned patients recovering from surgery in ER
are sometimes sent up here.)

During every other cycle there's a Code Blue
followed by a patient being wheeled out on their bed
with a white sheet pulled over their head.
The staff tries to move them discreetly, but I notice.

Last night, I heard a strange sound
coming from the room next door.

Curious, I crept out in my pajamas,
dragging my IV pole with me.

There was Death bent over an old woman,
his face close to hers, almost in a kiss.
Startled, Death glared at me, twisted his face into a rictus grin,
held his index finger to his black lips,
and slowly shook his head side to side.

Terrified, I hurried to my room, closed the door,

climbed beneath the blankets, trembling like a frightened child

hiding from a monster slouching darkly from the closet.

PITY PARTY

When my wife married me, I was strong, muscular, confident.
You could tell I had once been a body builder.

But six months of chemo stole that from me.
Nowadays, I'm gaunt, boney, withered—
a wasteland of flesh and blood.
When you look up "emaciated" in the dictionary
it shows a picture of me.

Before cancer, my hair was white and my blue eyes
sparkled with life. But now I am bald and wrinkly
like one of those hairless cats.

Chemo has made me ugly, turned me into something
I don't recognize.

I worry my wife won't want me anymore. Who would?
I know she vowed for better or for worse,
in sickness and in health, but I'm pretty sure
she didn't bargain on being hitched to a corpse.

AS I LAY DYING

Lately, it feels as if Death is squeezing my heart
in his boney grip, wringing the life out of it.

All day yesterday,
I felt like I might keel over and die at any time.

I was alone when suddenly I blacked out
and crumpled to the floor.

I imagined my wife and daughter finding me hours later,
rigored and dead as a doorknob.

My last thoughts before blackout were,
"This is it! This is what it's like to die."

Death is like that sometimes—
lonely as a sailor's ghost at the bottom of the sea.

SUBLIMINAL MAN

What I tell my wife:

If I die from cancer, I want you to be happy.

Time will dull the pain of losing me.

You'll grieve for a year or so,

but you'll move on. You need to move on.

I want you to love and to be loved.

Life is better when you share it with someone.

Just remember how much I loved you.

What I really think:

I can't die from this stupid cancer!

If I do, you'll meet another guy.

You'll live with him or get married and sleep together.

I don't want another man to see you naked.

I want to be the one who gets to touch and kiss you.

He'll get all the love I ever dreamed of.

I'd kick his ass if I wasn't dead.

BETWEEN DOUBT & FAITH

I never prayed to God

to cure me of my cancer. Not once.

After all—so the argument goes—

if God gave me cancer in the first place

who am I to plead for it to be taken away?

But now, close to the end of my chemotherapy,

it dawned on me that every person

who helped to create my cancer treatment

may have been put here intentionally.

When they were young, God might have instilled

their interest in science and medicine

and helped them get into colleges and universities.

Perhaps every meandering path in their lives

led them straight on their way to save me and others like me.

CHECKMATE

To pass time, I sometimes played chess during hospital stays.
Despite my chemo brain, I could still beat most challengers.

On the last day of six excruciating months of chemo,
Death comes and we play a game. It was the first time
I'd seen him since we ate churros in the desert.

Several times, he had me against the ropes,
but I fought back, captured all his pawns, killed his queen,
and chased his king into a corner.

"Checkmate!" I gloat, toppling his king. "You lose."

As a sullen Death departs, he stops and glares over his shoulder.

"You know, Johnny Boy," he hisses with his forked tongue.
"This isn't over. I'll be seeing you someday."
"Someday," I reply with a smirk as I do a little happy dance.
"But not today."

FOR WHOM THE BELL TOLLS

for Charlie C., Chuck E., Jim P., Amy S. & Carol B.

I got to ring the bell on the Oncology ward,

signaling that I'm all done, cancer-free. I'm going to live.

But some of my friends didn't make it.

Two died from cancer months before I was diagnosed.

A friend of the family recently passed after a stint in hospice.

Two thought their cancer had gone away,

but it returned with a vengeance.

All this brings me back to the questions I asked at the beginning:

"Why me? What did I do to deserve this?"

But the question is different now, full of survivor's guilt.

Why do I get to live and they do not? Why me?

I'm not special. They were loved as much as I am.

Instead of celebrating,

the bells that toll for them will be funeral bells.

BENEDICTION

for Steve M.

A month after I was cancer-free
I visited a preacher friend in Kansas City
who hadn't seen me during the six months
I was going through chemo.

We were sitting at a McDonalds having coffee
like we always do when I come to visit.

We joked about my baldness
and how I didn't have a strand of hair anywhere.

Before I left for the long drive home
we bowed our heads as my friend offered a prayer for my hair—

a hair prayer.

HOW TO SURVIVE CANCER

I barely made it through the punishing chemotherapy.

I'm still here—

wasted and weak, but here.

You want my advice on how to survive cancer?

Here it is:

Breathe in and out.

Don't die.

POETRY SAVED MY LIFE

Every day during my miserable bout with cancer,
I wrote poems about what I was going through.

My pockets were always crammed with scribbled notes
on scraps and pieces of paper.

During my hospitalizations and the time in between,
poetry was my constant companion.

I was never alone.

I wanted to live so I could share these poems
with people who might need them.

I wanted to live so I could teach my poetry class
and tell my students how poetry saved my life.

I wanted to live so you could read this poem
penned by a dying man during his darkest hours
by the dim, flickering light of a stub of melted candle.

HELP SPREAD THE WORD

If this book affected you or helped you in any way, please help spread the word. These poems deserve to be shared. Give this book as a gift to friends and relatives, young and old alike. Buy a copy for your local library. Write a book review for your local newspaper or church newspaper or newsletter, radio station, or favorite magazine. Write a review on amazon.com or on goodreads.com or elsewhere. Talk about it on Facebook. Tweet about it. Post a YouTube video or blog about it. Send an Instagram of the book cover. Ask your local librarian to recommend it. Ask your local bookseller to stock it. Discuss it in book clubs or in cancer patient/survivor support groups. Encourage its translation into other languages. The success of a book depends on readers like you who recommend it to their friends and others.

ABOUT THE POET

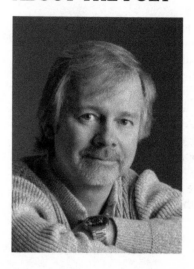

John Smelcer is the author of more than 60 books, including a dozen books of poetry. His most recent collection is *Raven*. His most recent nonfiction book is *Enacting Love: How Thomas Merton Died for Peace* (July 2022). For a quarter century, John was Poetry Editor at *Rosebud* Magazine, where he currently serves as Senior Editor Emeritus. From 2016-2020, he was the Inaugural Writer-in-Residence for the Charter for Compassion, the world's largest compassion movement with over five million members in 45 countries. Every April, during National Poetry Month, John teaches a global online course called "Poetry for Inspiration and Wellbeing." Nowadays, he is an official blogger for *Cure*, America's most widely read magazine for cancer patients, survivors, caretakers, and the people who love them. Learn more at www.johnsmelcer.com

Printed in the USA
CPSIA information can be obtained
at www.ICGtesting.com
CBHW032255090224
4213CB00001BA/49